Rhythm Healing:

PTSD, Trauma and Beyond

D. W. (Bill) Moore, LRT

SoulDance LLC

www.OutlawDrummers.com

Olympia, Washington U.S.A.

Copyright © by D.W. Moore

All right reserved. No part of this book may be reproduced in any form, except for brief reviews, without the permission of the Author.

Olympia, WA 98506 USA

Cover Art: © 2013 Bill Moore

ISBN 9781493706198

First Print, 2013

For more information:
www.OutlawDrummers.com
Bill@OutlawDrummers.com

Contents

Introduction...i

Chapter 1

The Neurology of Stress...1

Chapter 2

Elements of RMT

Cognitive Dissonance...10

Inclusion..13

Mindfulness Meditation...15

Reflexology..20

Imagery...21

Desensitization...23

Neuro- Linguistic Programming (NLP)..24

Social Synchronization and Entrainment...26

Binaural Beat Entrainment..28

Auditory Entrainment..30

Chapter 3

Empirical Effects of Drumming and Mindfulness Based Meditation

Telomeres..33

Cancer and Tumors..34

Genetic Markers..35

Chapter 4
Particulars about Different Groups
Social-emotional Behavior and Cognitive Development of Children……....38

Drug and Alcohol……………………………………………………...……42

Dementia/ Alzheimer's/Parkinson's ……………………………...………...43

Compassion Fatigue……………………………………………………..….45

PTSD……………………………………………………………………..…46

Soldiers…………………………………………………...…….…………..48

Team Building……………………………………………………………...50

Chapter 5
Healthcare Cost……………………………………………………………...52

Chapter 6
Social Change through Sound Community Psychology……………..……..54

Chapter 7
Summary……………………………………………………………………57

Appendix
A brief Overview of
RMT…………………………………………………………...……………61

Experiential Drumming………………………………………………….…..65

References……………………………………………………………………..70

Introduction

I grew up in a strict Christian family, but had so many questions that were not being answered by my pastor or my faith. I felt like there was so much more to the world and what was going on in it, which was being left out to me. My first experience in meditation came in 1976 during an Eckankar rally at Farragut State Park in North Idaho. I was working in the park that summer as part of a program called Youth Conservation Corp. Eckankar professed to be the science of soul travel. Although I didn't get involved with Eckankar, this really opened my eyes to new ways of thinking and particularly about meditation, which started giving me the tools to finding the answers that I was looking for. I studied and practiced meditation diligently for many years and felt like I was opening up a whole new world for myself. I was getting perspectives of the world that my friends and family didn't seem to understand, or want to know about. This caused conflict inside me; the excitement of learning new things and the pressure of wanting to be accepted in society caused me to put aside my meditation in the late 80's.

After participating in Desert Storm as a gunner on a Bradley Infantry Fighting Vehicle in the Army, my life started to go to pieces. My marriage was falling apart, I hated myself, I had no friends and my dreams terrified me so badly that I hated to go to sleep at night. I poured myself into my job as a pipefitter to try and divert my attention. I was too afraid to ask for help because of the stigma attached to soldiers with mental problems. I didn't want to be labeled "one of those people." After nearly going through with suicide, I realized that I needed a change. The only thing that had stopped my attempt at suicide was that my daughter had come home when I thought she was to be gone. I couldn't let her be the one to find me. This shocked me into a different path. I quit my job, got divorced, and moved back to North Idaho where I grew up. Right away I landed a job for one of the largest construction firms in the inland Northwest. They were just opening their new petroleum division. I applied for a foreman's position and ended up as the company's superintendant. Even though I put them in the black the first year, I was still not happy and was struggling with my personal life. Again I had buried myself in my work to cover the pain and anguish I was carrying. I just wanted it to stop.

Hand drumming came to me quite unexpectedly. I went to a dinner party with my roommate and got a drum put in front of me after dinner and was told to drum or leave. Since I was riding with my roommate (who had brought a drum), I stayed. To this day I still can't put words to the feeling that I felt after that encounter. It was very much like the meditation that I had known earlier in my life. My mind was much quieter and I was able to feel calmer. As some synchronicities can be in life, the next day I went to an arts and crafts fair. One of the performances was a West African style drum and dance troupe. I was blown away. I had never seen anything like it. I don't know why, but I turned to my roommate and told her that I was going to do that for the rest of my life. She started to laugh and told me that I needed to learn to drum first. I enrolled in drumming classes soon after. It was a struggle at first, but the feeling I felt afterwards was so much better than what I had been living with. I even started to meditate again. As I always do with everything I'm involved in, I started to pour myself into my meditation and studying drumming. Within a couple of years, I realized that my depression and anxiety had diminished considerably. I tried out for the local drum and dance troupe and got accepted. My drum teacher had me start teaching the new people in the class. He said it would be the best way for me to increase my own skills and give me greater balance. My students kept talking about how healing it felt. They would come into class talking about their weekly therapy session with their drums. This interested me that others seemed to be having a feeling of healing from the drums also. The drumming also got me acquainted with people working in the Mind-Body Medicine field. These people started introducing me to the connection between the mind and the body and gave me insights into new ways of thinking which had been very similar to what I had been discovering earlier in my life through my meditation. Between the drumming, being part of a group, and meditating, I started to get a whole new vision of myself and life. After five years with the troupe, it came to an end with everyone going their own ways in life. I and one of the dancers kept up the drum and dance classes in town. For the first time since the war, I was feeling stable and happy.

    I knew I needed to take the next step in my life, but was too afraid to make that step. Like most people, giving up the stability of a doing the job I knew, for making the changes that I wanted to see in my life felt, daunting. That next step came when I had scaffolding collapse at work and crushed a vertebra in my back. As I lay waiting for the ambulance, I realized that this was the turning point for me that I had been asking for, but I had not expected it to be quite as dramatic as this. One of my mentors had told me that you can't change what happens to you in your life, but our true power comes from changing our perception of it. Rather than taking this as another problem, I decided to take it as a blessing. My caretakers thought I must have hit my head also because any time anyone asked me about my accident, I would respond with what a blessing it was going to be for me. Yes, I still had the mental and physical struggles but I held on to that belief through the whole ordeal. My friends would pick me up and take me to the beach each week to watch the West African style dance classes that I had been drumming for, before the accident. The drummers would play and the dancers would dance around me. I would feel the rhythm in my healing body. Within two weeks, I was off of the pain medication and at the end of three months I was back working again. My doctors were astounded at my recovery. They had told me that I would be in pain the rest of my life because there was no real fix for this type of crushed vertebra: the doctor was wrong. I am now living that blessing that I had held as a positive belief and have no residual pain from my injury. I believe that our life is not determined by what happens to us; it is determined by the perception we perceive of it.

Chapter 1

The Neurology of Stress

As medical costs are going up and become increasingly unsustainable, new forms of cheaper proven healing modalities are needed. People with PTSD, trauma, and mood disorders have been proven to have damage in vital regions of the brain. These regions control all chemical and electrical impulses in the body. This damage prevents proper functioning and is caused by, or aggravated by stress. Stress seems to be a leading contributor to all disease of the mind and body. Stress can be created both physically and psychologically. It only makes sense that stress should be the focus of our healing. Also, quantum physics tells us that we are all just vibrations. Vibrations are a steady rhythm. Shouldn't that be the tool we use to heal?

By combining rhythm and meditation, there is overwhelming empirical evidence to show it to be a true healing modality rather than just a complementary or alternative medicine. This healing modality has been shown to be effective for the healing of PTSD, trauma, mood disorders, slows down Alzheimer's, dementia, Parkinson's disease, relieves drug and alcohol dependency, modifies social-emotional behavior and development in children, and can help fight cancer and tumors.

Throughout this book, I will be looking at what stress is, how it affects the body, and how by combining rhythm and meditation, we can target specific neural regions of the brain to do more than just stabilize the damage, but reverse a lot of the damage that is done from mild to severe chronic stress.

What is Stress and How Does It affect our Bodies and Minds?

In the on-line Oxford dictionary, stress is defined as "a state of mental or emotional strain or tension resulting from adverse or demanding circumstances." Most people understand what physical stress does, but we don't seem to realize that psychological stress means more than just traumatic events. People in our "modern" society don't seem to understand that we create stress and trauma from our own thoughts. We worry about everything. This worry creates the same reaction in our bodies that traumatic events cause. The mind doesn't know the difference; it just reacts. A little stress is good, but when this reaction goes on for long periods of time, it starts to cause damage to our minds and our bodies. Psychoneuroimmunology is the current science that is primarily looking at the interrelation between the mind and body. Research in this field has found that stress is a major contributor to how our bodies and minds function. They are not separate systems; they are a continuous feedback loop between the two. What happens to one, directly affects the other.

There are two major systems in the body which deal with stress, the sympathetic system and the parasympathetic system. The sympathetic system kicks in when we perceive a stressful situation. This is known as the fight or flight mode. The parasympathetic system resumes functioning normally after the perceived stress is over and this helps the body recover from the effects caused by the sympathetic system. Our bodies need both systems to function properly to stay healthy. If the sympathetic system continues for too long and we do not counter it with the parasympathetic system, damage occurs in the regulatory system of our body. This damage starts a downward chain of damage throughout the whole body.

Robert Sapolsky, in his book *Why Zebras Don't Get Ulcers,* looks at how psychological turmoil can cause us to be sick, speed up our aging process, make us vulnerable to depression, affect our memory, and even define where we stand on the social ladder (p. 3-4, 2004). In an evidence review titled "Post-Traumatic Stress Disorder: Evidence-Based Research for the Third Millennium," the researchers state, "The perception of stress leads to a significant load upon physiological regulation, including circadian regulation, sleep and psychoneuroendocrine-immune interaction" (2005). The sympathetic and the parasympathetic systems both have a lot to do with the healing your body gets. Too much of our sympathetic system (stress) and our bodies begin to perceive this mental state as the norm, causing more and more damage, leaving the body without its capability to self regulate. This is just like the now famous work in operant conditioning that Ivan Pavlov experimented with using his dogs and a bell. When a stressful occurrence happens over and over again for long periods, our minds and bodies react as if the sympathetic system running all the time is our normal state of being. Then, the parasympathetic system can feel like it is out of place. In other words, we forget what calm actually feels like and become uncomfortable in a calm, restful situation. When this happens, we need to learn how to calm ourselves down on a regular basis and condition ourselves into letting that be part of our norm again.

As our brains have evolved, we have come to the point of contemplating our past and our future. This contemplation can create some types of stress. "Essentially, we humans live well enough and long enough, and are smart enough, to generate all sorts of stressful events purely in our heads" (Sapolsky, p. 4, 2004). We worry about the future and regret our pasts; neither can we do anything about. This can cause the same type of stress caused by physical damage to the body. Again, our bodies don't know the difference. Because of our fast paced lives, we neglect our recovery time; our body needs that recovery time (allostasis). Allostasis is about letting the parasympathetic system take over and allowing the brain to process and coordinate stress relieving changes in the body and mind. Small amounts of the parasympathetic being activated in our lives can do big things for reversing that damage.

When we go into fight or flight mode, which can be triggered by any psychological, physical, or social disruption, our sympathetic nervous system kicks into action, dumping epinephrine and noreprinephrine into our systems to react to the emergency. At the same time, our parasympathetic system slows down to divert extra energy to the situation (Sapolsky, p.22-23, 2004). The body shuts down the function of some organs and increases others, dumping more hormones into the body. If we take the time after the emergency to calm down, our parasympathetic system returns to a stable state, the sympathetic system returns to normal and chemical allostasis is achieved. If we spend too much time in stressful situations, our bodies and minds can be damaged by these excessive hormones in the system, creating more stress and more disease. This continued stress can rewire our brains into believing that this is the norm and begin a vicious cycle of damage. Sapolsky compares us to zebras which go through their fight or flight mode, but take the time to rest, relax, and not worry about what has been or could be, which allows the body and mind to heal. We have lost this in our fast paced, stress filled lives. People with PTSD find that this continuous running of our sympathetic system can become a self sustaining feedback loop and can imprint in our neural network until "the symptoms become increasingly entrenched, and often worsen" (Naparstek, p. 77, 2006).

The amygdala is one part of the brain that is first to decide if you are in a stressful situation. "So the aroused amygdala activates the sympathetic nervous system and, an aroused sympathetic nervous system increases the odds of the amygdala activating. Anxiety can feed itself" (Sapolsky, p. 322, 2004). "PET scans and recent research have shown how traumatic events leave distinctive footprints on the brain" (Naparstek, p. 157, 2006).

At the base of the brain is the hypothalamus. The hypothalamus contains hormones that control the pituitary which "in turn regulates the secretion of the peripheral glands" (Sapolsky, p. 29). When we encounter a stressful situation, the hypothalamus kicks into action and releases hormones into the adrenal glands which causes a release of glucocorticoids into our body. "Together, glucocorticoids and the secretions of the sympathetic nervous system (epinephrine and noreprinephrine) account for a large percentage of what happens in your body during stress" (Sapolsky, p. 31-32, 2004). A little of this is good for the body, but extended stress can have dire consequences. Axons and dendrites can actually start shrinking and pulling apart, thereby reducing the effectiveness of the neural network (Sapolsky, p. 217, 2004). This extended stress has a reaction that has effects upon our cardiovascular system, neural system, metabolism, appetite, bowel function, gastrointestinal function, blood pressure, skeletal growth, sex and reproductive systems, immunity, and pain response, just to name a few. It also causes neurological connection damage to the hippocampus which causes memory problems (Sapolsky, p. 215, 2004). In chronic PTSD patients, it was found that cortisol levels actually drop below normal levels and then during stressors, peak dramatically and then fall back below normal again afterwards (Naparstek, p. 62-63, 2006). Sapolsky goes on to say that "people with PTSD from repeated trauma (as opposed to single trauma)--soldiers exposed to severe carnage in combat, individuals repeatedly abused as children--have smaller hippocampus" (p. 221, 2004). He also says that "prolonged major depression is, once again, associated with a smaller hippocampus" (p. 221, 2004). What is still in question in some circles is whether the smaller hippocampus came before or after the trauma. He does say that in studies of Cushing's syndrome, it gives us hints into which came first; that if you stop the glucocorticoids excess, the neurons in the hippocampus begin to regrow (p. 222-223, 2004). Either way, the hippocampus can be increased in size, which is the main point. "Of course, challenging mental activities will increase the likelihood that our hippocampal neurons will survive" (Doidge, p. 256, 2007); although, any new mental activity helps. Learning new things builds new neural pathways.

    I would like to use mechanical metaphors for the body, even though our bodies are so much more complex, because it will give you a better visualization. In your car, if the battery isn't allowing enough sparks to the engine, the car runs lousy. If the fuel is not getting to your engine properly, the car runs lousy. Like our cars, the body has an amazing feedback system. "The body can not only sense something stressful, but it also is amazingly accurate at measuring just how far and how fast that stressor is throwing the body out of allostatic balance"

(Sapolsky, p. 253, 2004). The thing to look at here is that if the parts of our brain that control our electrical and chemical impulses in the body are damaged, the whole system starts to break down. This is the root of why we start having problems in our minds and our bodies. Western medicine seems to only be looking at the symptoms and the relief of those symptoms. Kabat-Zinn calls it a "disease care system," not a health care system (2011). Any true healing form needs to work with the root problem, not just the symptoms.

What is now being looked at for true healing in the body is how our thoughts can actually have a modulating effect on our bodies. The biggest difference found in how some people cope with stress better than others is how they perceive and appraise their stress, and how they react to their stress (Sapolsky, p. 254, 2004). Sapolsky gives five things that can be done to modulate stress within the body. First is finding an outlet for our frustration, second is social support, third is predictability, fourth is control of our environment, and lastly is a perception that things are getting better (p. 255-263, 2004). These main points are also made throughout the Mind-Body field in different forms. By combining drumming and meditation into one modality, we can cover all these points and more, to reduce and reverse the effects of the sympathetic system and help the parasympathetic system work to optimum efficiency to recover the body to allostasis. Rhythm Meditation Therapy (RMT) targets specific neural functions to create new neural pathways around the damaged portions of the brain. RMT also targets the five points Sapolsky mentioned; it gives an outlet for frustration and anger in a healthy, creative way. It also allows us to gather together for social support. The setting of a steady rhythm gives us a steady form of predictability. During the drumming, we also have control over our part of the rhythm; each person putting in what they feel that they can. Social support can also help us feel that things are not as bad as they feel when we are alone and isolated. Doing this on a regular basis changes our operant conditioning back to a more stabilized self-sustaining state. This is a good point for our healing journey to begin.

Chapter 2

Elements of RMT

Cognitive Dissonance

I showed earlier that Sapolsky made the statement that our own inner dialogue can cause us as much stress as a physical trauma event. Self help books talk about the power of positive thinking. I had tried the power of positive thinking before in my life and found that it lacked something. I found that we can't just consciously say "I'm healed, I'm healed," because there is the subconscious part of us inside calling "Bullshit." Our subconscious knows it's not true, no matter how much the conscious part of us wants to insert itself. This causes dissonance within ourselves and slows down any healing process.

Encyclopedia Britannica defines cognitive dissonance as: "the mental conflict that occurs when beliefs or assumptions are contradicted by new information. The unease or tension that the conflict arouses in a person is relieved by one of several defensive maneuvers: the person rejects, explains away, or avoids the new information, persuades himself that no conflict really exists, reconciles the differences, or resorts to any other defensive means of preserving stability or order in his conception of the world and of himself." This dissonance creates a dilemma which leads us to possibly change our perception, choose to ignore what we see right in front of us, or completely reject that it ever happened.

Our subconscious has the power to only see what it chooses to see even if overwhelming evidence says otherwise.

    Because our lives need to be about accepting what is, we first have to accept and embrace what has happened and then frame the healing for our future. My mantra through my whole experience with my crushed vertebra was "I accept what is happening to me right here, right now, and know that it will be to my benefit in the future." This change in thought had dramatic effects upon my physical body. No more dissonance. This was similar to what I had been using for my recovery from my mental and physical issues from my trauma from the war. I had to accept that it happened and reframe my perception from "poor me" to looking at it as a learning experience that I never could have had in any other way. This opened something up inside me, which led to growth and a long road of recovery. I was later to learn that this was part of what is now called "mindfulness." Mindfulness is about living in the present moment, the here and now. It is about getting away from the fear and regret of the past and also staying out of the fear of the future which you can't control anyway.

    Our focus determines our reality. If we focus on the past fears and pain or focus on what might be, that is what will come to us. By staying in the here and now and finding something in our reasoning to be grateful for *right here, right now*, that becomes our reality. We get more to be grateful for. In my research into stress related disease, I came across two leading neurologists and many Buddhist practitioners who say the same thing. It felt good to find validation from some of the top minds in the world.

While in the navy, straight out of high school, I met a Navy Seal who gave me new perspective on how to deal with pain. He told me that if you reject the pain it comes back harder, but if you can find something inside yourself to accept the pain, it will leave quicker. For every action, there is an equal and opposite reaction. He told me that he always looked at pain as just the messenger to tell you that you were hurt and to not reject the messenger. By thanking the messenger for its wonderful message over and over again, we can change how our body reacts to the injury. I have found over the years that this is not as easy as it sounds, but it does work and we can train ourselves to get better and better at it all the time. This method is not simple, but it is long lasting. When I crushed my vertebra in my back, I used this method and was completely off of pain killers in two weeks and out of chronic pain in a month. I now live pain free even though the doctors told me I would have pain the rest of my life. I watched my father get hooked on prescription pain killers for injuries he had received in an accident. I did not want to be one of those pill poppers just to get through each day. Again, the power of the mind over the body without dissonance is where our true power lies.

From the time I was little, I was told that true power, health, and happiness comes from something outside myself and that as long as I pursued that, I could be happy and healthy. Through my whole journey in this world, the most profound thing that I have learned, is that true healing of the mind and the body comes from within us and not from outside ourselves. Not to say that Western medicine doesn't have a place in healing, but we need a balance of both to get us from the damage done, back to a balanced whole person again. We have to take a holistic view; look at the whole picture. Sometimes Western medicine is needed to stabilize us from the mental or physical damage that has occurred in our lives, and then we need to look at our perception of that damage and make different choices of how to perceive the damage. This is what gets us on the road back to balanced health. Mental cognative dissonance slows or stops the healing process.

Inclusion

The reason for group therapy is to create inclusion and social support. I have worked with people from ages 5 to 93, all genders, disabled and non-disabled. All could participate at their own level and be included in the process of creating something together. At one drum circle I attended, there was a man in his 90's who just added one steady down beat because that was all he said he was capable of doing. During a break he commented that he didn't feel that he was making a difference in the group. I suggested that when the group started up again, he start like he normally would, but after about a minute or so, he should stop. He gave me a quizzical look but agreed to try this. The next round of playing, he started as usual, and then suddenly stopped after about a minute. The whole group wavered for a second before it restabilized and every head in the group came up. The elderly gentleman got the biggest grin on his face because of the reaction by the entire group. He knew that what little he was doing did made a difference. "Even in our obsessively individualistic society, most of us yearn to feel part of something larger than ourselves" (Sapolsky, p. 416, 2004).

    Our self esteem is at the root of who we are and how we perceive ourselves in society. Self esteem (also called self-worth, self-confidence, and self respect) reflects a person's self appraisal of their own value in society. Sapolsky also says that people with a support system have less cardiovascular stress responses and have a three times better survival rate than those without a support system (p. 257-258, 2004). "Equally important, our self-esteem is bound up in this ability to impact our world" (Naparstek, p. 39, 2006). In Anne Harington's book, *The Cure Within*, she found by looking at a nine year long database, that people with social support lived longer than those without "...even after factors such as socioeconomic status, smoking, alcohol use, obesity, physical activity, and use of preventive health services were accounted for" (p. 184, 2008). The World Health Organization did a three decade long study that showed similar outcomes. They found that social support was a "major and important role in the outcome of disease" (Mehl-Madrona, p. 39, 2007). We are social creatures, who when damaged emotionally and physically pull away from others, which is counterproductive to our health. "People with PTSD can become quite secretive and opaque, going to great lengths to avoid any feelingful connection, because feelings of any sort are so overwhelming and painful (Naparstek, p.129, 2006).

RMT is non-threatening. You are allowed to participate at any level which feels comfortable to you. You are not asked to do anything more than sit, listen and breathe if that is all you can allow yourself to do and you will still benefit. It is good to reassure clients that they only have to participate if they feel drawn, because many people are intimidated by the drums and think that it takes skill to master it, or just don't want to do anything. This anxiety can create more problems if not set to the side before you start. "Fear is an element that prevents us from letting go. We're fearful that if we let go we'll have nothing else to cling to. Letting go is a practice; it's an art" (Hanh, p.25, 2009). Meditation helps to look at those fears and learn what to do with them in a safe and non-invasive way.

Mindfulness Meditation

Many people have the wrong perception of meditation. They assume that it is about clearing the mind. I personally have never met anyone who can do that. That is the reason I found mindfulness meditation to be so helpful. It is not about clearing your mind, but about paying attention to the present moment and whatever that may bring up. When you find yourself drifting away from the present, thank the thought that came into your mind, without judgment of yourself or the thought, and come back to the present. "You have to train yourself, to learn how to go home to the present moment, to the here and now, and to take care of that moment, to take care of your body and your feelings in this moment. That is the most effective way to deal with anxiety or worries" (Hanh, p. 152, 2009). "Mindfulness is the capacity to recognize what is there without being attached to it or fight and suppress it" (Hanh, p. 26, 2009). Leading neurologist Jon Kabat-Zinn says it is not about trying to get somewhere, but about just simply being aware in this present moment (2011). Sapolsky talks about meditation as a way of healing. "When done on a regular basis (that is to say, something close to daily, for fifteen, thirty minutes at a time), meditation seems to be pretty good for your health, decreases glucocorticoid levels, sympathetic tone, and all the bad stuff that too much of either can cause" (p. 402, 2004). Meditation in one form or another has been used down through the recorded history of humans and has the longest history of recorded healing results. We are just now being able to see empirical results through new brain imagery devices.

Jon Kabat-Zinn, in his lecture on "The Healing Power of Mindfulness," says that along with accepting what is and not judging it, and reframing our perception of the trauma, we also need to recognize the beauty within ourselves that already exists (2011). His research into mindfulness has shown that it increases the lengths of our telomeres (the end cap on our genes), thins down the amygdala, and increases the size of the left frontal cortex which is known through EEG's to have something to do with approach and emotional balance (2011). Being present may sound simple, but Kabat-Zinn says that it is a skill like any other that needs be learned and worked at. Part of that involves looking at fear when it does present itself in your present, looking at it without the judgment and just being aware of it (2011). It sounds easy, but takes your will to change old ways of doing things and viewing things; one step at a time.

Thich Nhat Hanh in his book *Answers from the Heart* says that when fear arises, we need to only recognize it and its strength will be lost. "If it comes back again, you do it again, and it will continue to lose its strength. You don't have to fight it, just recognize and smile at it. Every time you recognize it, it becomes weaker until eventually it can't control you anymore (p. 19-20, 2009). He also says that, "You have to be one hundred percent in the here and now (p. 18, 2009). "Handling the present moment with all your attention, all your intelligence, is already building a future" (p. 19, 2009). Robert Sapolsky, another leading neurologist, in his book *Why Zebras Don't Get Ulcers*, says the same thing; "…it can be stress-reducing to merely admit that you're hurting emotionally from the stressor" (p. 411, 2004).

Even the U.S. Department of Veterans Affairs has done research into mindfulness type treatments. Their conclusion is that "Mindfulness-based approaches have been shown to be useful for problems commonly seen in trauma survivors such as anxiety and hyperarousal. Mindfulness practice has potential to be of benefit to individuals with PTSD, either as a tertiary or a stand-alone treatment" (Vujanovic, Niles, Pietrefesa, Potter, & Schmertz, 2011).

In a Buddhist Psychotherapy class, I was taught that we cannot control what happens to us in life; good things happen and bad things happen. The only thing we can control is our perception of it. This fits with other teachings that I have learned. Basic science teaches us that for every action there is an equal and opposite reaction. If we take that into consideration in healing, we find that the more we *reject* what happened to us, the more damage is created in our bodies. It is when we can accept what happens to us and embrace these changes that things begin to change. We are all taught that if you can just be healthy, you can be happy. What I have learned is that if you can be happy, then you can be healthy. Most people reject that idea because it is the harder path to take and is not the instant fix that they want. The instant fix doesn't really last though. It is all an illusion which leads to more and more problems down the road. It is when you can find the strength to make the hard decisions and work toward changing physical and mental patterns that permanent changes begin to happen. The only time you can drum with anyone is in the present moment. You can't drum with someone in the future and you can't drum with someone in the past. We all learn in one or two of three ways, either auditory, visually, or kinesthetically. By bringing all three representation systems into the here and now, it is possible to entrain our whole minds in the here and now and away from getting caught in the past or the future. This goes back to operant conditioning; training ourselves to stay present. We can't do anything about the past or the future, so our attention needs to be here and now where we can do something about our present moment. A quote that is often attributed to Albert Einstein is "Insanity is doing the same thing over and over again but expecting different results." If what you are currently doing is not working, try something else.

Reflexology

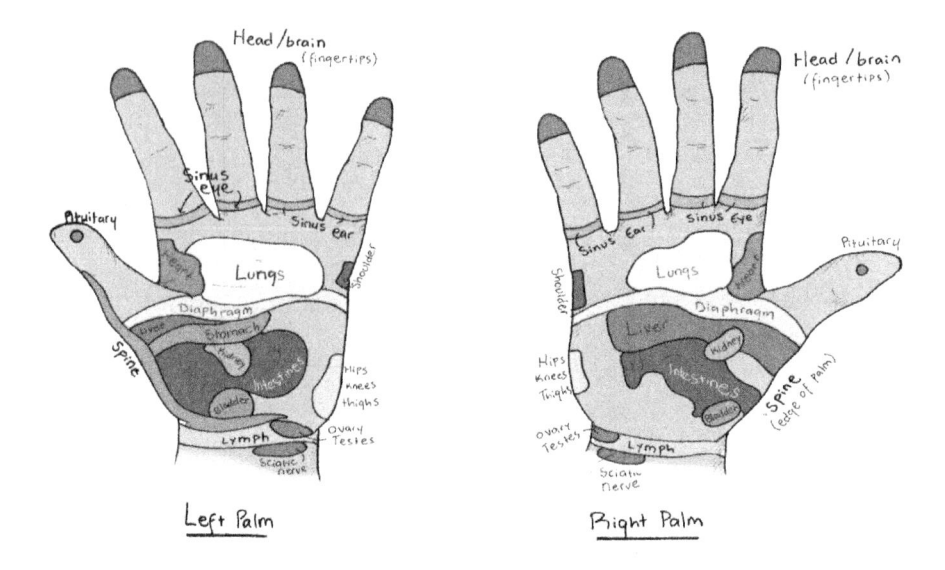

Left Palm   *Right Palm*

Although the practice of reflexology has been around for thousands of years, modern practices are based on research into "nervous reflex actions" that were studied over a hundred years ago (Crane, p. 14, 1998). Reflexology is about manipulating nerve endings in the hands and/or the feet to help restore balance in the autonomic system, which includes the sympathetic and the parasympathetic systems of the body (Crane, p. 20, 1998). For this book, we will be looking at how tapping on the edge of the drum stimulates the nerve systems in our hands. Each nerve system in our bodies circulates through our hands. Drumming can also stimulate these points and help the body to kick in the parasympathetic system to bring the body to homeostasis. The journal article Effect of Reflexology on EEG – A Nonlinear Approach states "…reflexological stimulation, from the signals and systems point of view, brings the brain–mind mechanism to a lower dimensional chaos indicating a state of 'order out of disorder" (Kannathal, Paul, Lim, & Chua, p. 649, 2004). Sala Horowitz, in her article "Evidence Based Reflexology" shows that reflexology can decrease lower back pain and the pain caused during cancer treatment (Horowitz, p. 215, 2004). Bringing in the stimulation of the hands adds another dimension to the healing process of RMT. More can be added to the session if you choose to have the clients tap up and down the length of the palms of their hands on the edge of the drum.

I started doing foot reflexology in the 1970's to help my mother with her bursitis in her elbows. I was skeptical about its capabilities at first, but over the years I have found that reflexology of the feet or hands can be a very non-invasive way of getting the body back into homeostasis where it can heal itself.

Imagery

Using imagery is another distinctive modality that I have incorporated into RMT because of its proven ability to make psychological, emotional, and physical changes in people with stress and trauma issues. "Guided imagery is a form of deliberate, directed daydreaming—a purposeful use of the imagination, using words and phrases designed to evoke rich, multisensory fantasy and memory, in order to create a deeply immersive, receptive mind state that is ideal for catalyzing desired changes in mind, body, psyche, and spirit" (Naparstek, p. 149, 2006). The "two cerebral hemispheres of the brain in humans serve different functions" (Bandler & Grinder, p. 12, 1975). Belleruth Naparstek points out in her book *Invisible Heroes: Survivors of Trauma and How They Heal* that accessing only the left portion of the brain, which deals with the analytical and logical side of us, doesn't help, and can actually retraumatize the individual. "If a deeply traumatized person is prompted *only* to speak and think about the event that created his distress, without enlisting help from the imaginal, emotional, sensory, and somatic capabilities of his right brain, his symptoms can actually get worse instead of better" (Naparstek, p. XVIII, 2006). "This is because the language centers in the brain have been impaired by a cascade of biochemical responses, set loose by our built in, biologically driven, survival reactions during the time of the traumatic event itself" (p. XVIII, 2006). I have heard the same thing from several therapists that I have worked with over the years. Talk therapy has a tendency to retraumatize rather than help. Imagery accesses the right hemisphere of the brain and bypasses the left hemisphere's influence. "The primitive brain and midbrain cannot process cognitive solutions aimed at the higher cortical functions. But imagery, with its calming voice tones, soothing music and symbolic representations of safety, can settle down hypervigilant brain functioning and allow the brain to get back to doing its job" (Naparstek, p. 157, 2006). These new techniques are being developed to work with the brain in its own healing rather than against the brain and causing deeper trauma. Bandler and Grinder tell us that by accessing the creative portions of the brain, we open potential which is not normally experienced (p. 60-61, 1975). They also go on to say that we need to use all our representation systems (visual, auditory, kinesthetic) to achieve fuller experience (p. 137, 1975). Using RMT, the visual is achieved through the guided imagery, the auditory is accessed through the sound of the rhythm and the voice, and the kinesthetic is achieved through the hands on the drum and through the breathing of the individual.

Desensitization

Many soldiers and others with PTSD have hyper sensitization to sights, sounds, and images. In a war zone, soldiers have to keep every sense running on high all the time to keep themselves and their buddies alive. Because of this extreme heightened use, this hypersensitivity becomes the operant conditioning. Using RMT, soldiers can establish new responses to this wartime conditioning.

After Desert Storm, I had no idea that things which had been everyday life to me before would set my nerves on edge when I got home. I couldn't walk anywhere without subconsciously watching closely where I walked, or checking people's hands for weapons. I was constantly looking for safe places to hide. Loud noises would make me cringe. The 4th of July was not a day of celebration, but a day of nerve wracking stress, which I couldn't wait to get past. Night time gave me no relief. Every night, wondering in the back of my mind if I will wake in the morning. My dreams kept me waking all night, soaked in sweat. I would put off going to sleep at night so I didn't have that to deal with. Lack of sleep was pushing me closer to the edge. I started to believe that killing myself was the only way out for me.

Mindfulness meditation helped me to start being in the here and now rather than always worrying what might be ahead of me. It helped me realize that this new war zone was only in my own head. The tapping of the drums helped me disassociate the sounds around me from gunfire and explosions. It allowed me to control the sounds in a safe creative way. Drumming, breathing and meditation helped me to let go of the frustrations, anger and aggressions of the day so that I could actually sleep through the night. Slowly the nightmares diminished. I don't think that I will ever be 100% back to where I was before. I can't deny where I have been, but where I am now is so much better than where I was.

Neuro-Linguistic Programming (NLP)

NLP is a form of hypnosis which uses linguistic phrases to modify behavior. You don't have to put someone in an altered state to get reactions from the individual. It is a way of speaking to elicit responses. Mainstream medicine has not accepted it as a solid science yet, but advertisers and marketing personnel find it to be one of their primary tools. Here there is a fine line between ethical and unethical use. When used ethically, it can be a great tool to help individuals start to look at things from a different perspective. Psychoneuroimmunology has found that what we think has direct effects upon our body and mind. As shown before, our own inner dialog can be very unhealthy for us.

In research done by Richard Bandler and John Grinder, they noticed that by the way they phrased things they could elicit predictable responses from people; not just the wording, but also how it was being said. "Altered tone of voice can constitute an actual vocabulary of transformation of verbal communication, as can body language" (Bandler & Grinder, p. viii, 1975). They also found that by listening to subjects, they could establish how that person processed things in their mind. Everyone learns from visual, auditory, or kinesthetic stimulus. Some people use a combination of two of these. By listening to what is said, such as I *see* what you are saying, I *hear* what you are saying, or I *understand* what you are saying, we can get clues to how that person learns and can respond back in their learning form. This helps that person process what you are saying better. Bandler and Grinder named this process pacing. We must first understand how someone views their world before we can show them new ways of viewing the world. No two people view the world in the same way. This full process in hypnosis is called pacing and leading. "A hypnotist has successfully paced a client verbally when the hypnotist's verbalizations are accepted by the client as an accurate description of the client's ongoing experience" (Bandler & Grinder, p. 15, 1975). From that point you can start adding in therapeutic suggestions which can alter the client's internal dialog to a healthier way of thought; this is the leading. The tapping on the drum at the same time anchors these suggestions in the subconscious. In a quote from famed hypnotist Milton H. Erickson, they state "Hypnosis is essentially a communication of ideas and understandings to a patient in such a fashion that he will be more receptive to the presented ideas and thereby be motivated to explore his own body potentials for the control of his psychological and physiological responses and behaviors" (Bandler & Grinder, p. 179, 1975). I must caution the readers to understand that this technique should not be used without formal training. Unintended verbal cues could just as easily cause more damage to the client as it could to help the client.

Social Synchronization and Entrainment

Christine Stevens, in her book *Music Medicine* defines entrainment as a "synchronization of separate rhythms" (p. 31, 2012). Our bodies and minds are all affected by these synchronizations such as sleeping and waking with night and day, or the rhythm of a woman's menstrual cycle to the lunar cycle. (p. 31, 2012). Drumming can also create synchronization between people. "Humans are the only primates that spontaneously synchronize their voices and movements during music making and dancing, a behavior found across all cultures and emerging early in human childhood" (Kokal et al., 2011).

Entrainment through drumming is more than just getting people to synchronize together in the dominant beat. Entrainment can synchronize people in a group to a shared state of being. It helps people feel a connection to those around them and also has the capability of synchronizing our brain's molecular energy. Robert Friedman goes into depth about hemispheric synchronization in his book *The Healing Power of the Drum*; he talks about how our two hemispheres of our brain don't normally work together at the same time and can also have separate frequencies. "The right brain functions as the creative, visual, aural and emotional center. The left brain is the rational, logical, analytical and verbal administrator" (p.45, 2000). He also states that through "hemispheric synchronization," we can encourage our minds to work better (p. 45, 2000). "A decrease in trait anxiety occurred, reflecting an improvement in the participant's perceived reaction and ability to cope with stress and anxiety in general" (Wahbeh, Calabrese, & Zwickey, 2007). This synchronization can be achieved through rhythm. "As the two hemispheres begin to resonate to a single rhythm, a sense of clarity and heightened awareness arises. The individual is able to draw on both the left and the right hemispheres simultaneously. The mind becomes sharper, more lucid, synthesizing much more rapidly than normal, and emotions are easier to understand and transform (p. 45, 2000). Music has been shown in neurological studies to have no central region of the brain (Baeck, 2002). It takes both hemispheres working together to process music. This is what makes music different than any other stimulus. Most everything else has a particular region of the brain that is affected by that certain stimulus. "People suffering from cognitive functioning deficits, stress, pain, headache/migraines, PMS, and behavioral problems benefited from BWE (brain wave entrainment)" (Huang & Charyton, 2008).

Binaural Beat Entrainment

During my research into how sound and rhythm affect the human body, I came across research being done into binaural beat entrainment. This has to do with putting one frequency into one ear and another frequency into the other ear. The brain then builds a third frequency which gaps the difference between the two frequencies, creating a sound only heard within your own mind (Kasprzak, 2011). "For example, mixing tones of 100 Hz and 110 Hz yields a signal with a perceived frequency of 105 Hz that rises and falls in amplitude with a frequency of 10 Hz" (Lane, Kasian, Owens, & Marsh, 1998). Lane and his associates also state that "Results suggest that the presentation of binaural auditory beats can affect psychomotor performance and mood. This technology may have applications for the control of attention and arousal and the enhancement of human performance." Whether it is used for children or corporate staffs, this could mean an overall increase in learning and productivity.

On an EEG it was found that this sound decreases the alpha and beta amplitude while increasing the theta states of consciousness (Kasprzak, 2011). The theta brain wave state of consciousness is related to REM sleep.

> "Normal outward focused attention generates beta waves which vibrate from 14 to 40 cycles per second. When awareness shifts to an internal focus, our brain slows down into the rhythmical waves of alpha, vibrating at 7-14 waves per second. Alpha is defined by relaxation and centering. Dropping down to 4-7 cycles per second the brain enters the theta state in which there is an interfacing of conscious and unconscious process, producing hypnagogic dream-like imagery at the threshold of sleep. Theta is the source of sudden mystical insights and creative solutions to complex situations and is marked by physical and emotional healing. People with a preponderance of theta brainwaves are also able to learn and process much more information than normal" (Friedman, p. 44-45, 2000).

Although during drumming there are many sounds going in each ear, the description of the sound being created only inside our minds reminded me of an oral tradition which was passed down to me through West African drum teachers. When I first heard about what they called "ghost voices" or "ancestor voices," I thought it was a metaphor for something that I wasn't understanding. The first time I actually heard it, I realized it was not a metaphor, but a true sound created by the harmonics of the drums. I have heard the singing sounds many times now throughout my drumming experience since, with all different kinds of groups at various levels of drumming and thought that it would be interesting to mention because of the healing power of individual sounds compared to multiple sounds. It might be of interest for someone to actually do research into whether the sound heard during binaural beats has anything to do with the ghost voices from the oral African tradition.

I know that each time I have heard the singing, it has been around major transitions in my life. There are definite nonverbal reactions from everyone in the area of the occurrence; the look of surprise from those who are hearing it for the first time and the look of bliss on the faces of those who have heard the songs before. The closest I can describe it in relation to my religious background is the singing of angels from all directions at once; it feels like the sound surrounds you. It is a very surreal experience.

Auditory Entrainment

Hearing has been traditionally regarded as just a stimulus analyzer, but now, new research is finding that it is much more than that. A study by Norman Weinberger and his associate states, "studies of associative learning-induced plasticity in the primary auditory cortex (A1) indicate involvement in learning, memory and other cognitive processes. For example, the area of representation of a tone becomes larger for stronger auditory memories and the magnitude of area gain is proportional to the degree that a tone becomes behaviorally important. Here, we used extinction to investigate whether 'behavioral importance' specifically reflects a sound's ability to predict reinforcement (reward or punishment) vs. to predict any significant change in the meaning of a sound" (Bieszczad & Weinberger, p. 598, 2012). "These findings show that primary sensory cortical representation can encode behavioral importance as a signal's value to predict reinforcement, and that the number of cells tuned to a stimulus can dictate its ability to command behavior" (Bieszczad & Weinberger, p. 598, 2012). In simpler words, this means that when certain tonal frequencies are applied to a stimulus such as relaxation, the brain will assign brain function and cortical plasticity to this stimulus over the prior stimulus. This effect is what they are referring to as extinction; meaning to add priority in our minds for the new stimulus over prior stimulus. The frequencies which were used in these experiments to gain greater cortical plasticity are within the same frequency ranges that were seen in the binaural beat entrainment in the previous section. This shows further evidence of why the drums have such an effect upon neural changes within the mind. By adding greater importance in our minds to the new stimulus over a prior stimulus, we are creating stronger neural bonds to the new stimulus, thereby remembering them more clearly than the old stimulus. Anything we can do for people who have suffered trauma to help them create stronger bonds to good memories over bad memories can be significant for starting to truly heal.

Chapter 3
Empirical Effects of Drumming and Mindfulness Based Meditation

Telomeres

Telomeres are the end caps on our genes. Alzheimer's, dementia, Parkinson's disease, PTSD, and general mood disorder patients have all been reported to have smaller telomeres than average subjects, and these smaller telomeres lead to gene destabilization (Blackburn, Greider, & Szostak, 2006). Gene destabilization can also lead to premature aging and cognitive stress (Epel, Daubenmier, Moskowitz, Folkman, & Blackburn, 2009). Stress has been shown to be the main factor in the decrease of the size of telomeres (Epel et al., 2009). Because this is a stress related effect on the body, anything to do with stress relief can help with healing. The study "Can meditation slow rate of cellular aging? Cognitive stress, mindfulness, and telomeres" showed a direct effect of mindfulness meditation on telomere length (Epel et al., 2009). This research shows direct effects on our genetic system due to stress relief. As was shown earlier, drumming is an easy form of mindfulness meditation. You can't drum with someone in the future or the past, you can only drum with someone in the here and now. It seems to be such a simple concept to reduce our stress to increase our quality and length of life. But in our fast paced world, we don't take the time to simply sit, breathe, and be thankful for just a few moments in each day.

Cancer and Tumors

Dr. Barry Bittman and his research group looked into the effects of drumming on the neuroendocrine-immune parameters of the human body (Bittman, Berk, Felten, Westengard, Simonton, Pappas, & Ninehouser, 2001). What they found was that drumming didn't just slow down or stop damage done by stress to the human body, but it actually reversed several parameters tested. "These changes appear to be immunoenhancing (increased DHEA-to-cortisol ratios, increased NK cell activity, and increased LAK cell activity)" (Bittman et al.. p. 46, 2001). (DHEA) Dehydroepiandrosterone is a hormone that counteracts the presence of prolonged cortisol in our entire system. NK killer cells are cells that attack cancer in our bodies and LAK cells attack tumor cells. In this study, 111 age and sex matched non-prior drumming volunteers were a part of the research. This was to show that non drummers can be influenced by the drumming (Bittman et al., 2001). Any level of drumming can make these parameter changes; you don't have to be proficient at drumming to have changes occur. Bittman shows that for the drumming to be healing, it has to be put across in a non-threatening way. Many people are intimidated by trying to drum or play any musical instrument. Most instruments do need some type of proficiency to be able to play; but not drums. Anyone can play a drum at whatever level they are comfortable with, with no prior knowledge or experience, and get healing results. The trick is to get people past their anxiety about drumming. That is why I start people with just the right-left tapping and try to stay away from asking them to drum for the beginning of the Rhythm Meditation Therapy. Tapping seems to be okay with most people who would never try to drum with you. "I can't drum" is the response usually given, but most will just tap if the drum is in front of them already.

Genetic Markers

Since the genome project, scientists have started looking into genetic markers for disease control. They found that stress markers have a lot to do with the immune system. In a study called "Recreational music-making modulates the human stress response: a preliminary individualized gene expression strategy," Barry Bittman and his team used 45 immune response-related genes from participants blood to monitor the stress response during a one hour drumming session. "19 out of 45 markers demonstrated reversal with significant ($P=0.05$) Pearson correlations in contrast to 6 out of 45 markers in the resting control group and 0 out of 45 in the ongoing stressor group" (Bittman, Berk, Shannon, Sharaf,

Westengard, Guegler, & Ruff, 2005). Their conclusion was that drumming "warrants additional consideration as a rational choice within our armamentarium of stress reduction strategies." Drumming does more than stabilize or slow down stress response, it actually reverses damage done by stress at the genetic level. This is significant information when we are looking at ways of increasing our health and doing it in the most cost effective way. Modern medicine is known to usually only treat symptoms. True healing modalities must relieve symptoms and also reverse damage that has been done. That is the only way that you can start bringing clients off of the increasingly more expensive pharmaceuticals and back to homeostasis for the individual. Most pharmaceuticals are only made to stabilize, not to heal: a fact that the pharmaceutical companies don't want you to know. That is why they dominate the Continuing Medical Education (CME) of the health field.

> "Graduation from medical school and completion of residency training are the first steps in a career-long educational process for physicians. To take advantage of the growing array of diagnostic and treatment options, physicians must continually update their technical knowledge and practice skills. CME is a mainstay for such learning. Most State licensing authorities require physicians to complete a certain number of hours of accredited CME within prescribed timeframes to maintain their medical

licenses. Hospitals and other institutions may impose additional CME requirements upon physicians who practice at their facilities."

"Although some physicians pay the full expense of this additional education, more often the programs are either fully or partially subsidized by sponsors that provide educational grants and other funding to CME providers. Frequently, these sponsors are manufacturers of drugs, biologics, or medical devices related to the topic of the CME program."

"According to the Accreditation Council for Continuing Medical Education (ACCME), in 2007, the pharmaceutical industry spent more than a billion dollars to cover more than half the costs for CME activities conducted in the United States that year. Moreover, industry funding of accredited CME increased by more than 300 percent between 1998 and 2007" (Office of inspector general: Department of Health and Human Services, 2009).

This report goes on to say in its final conclusion, "There is growing concern about the integrity of medical education and the financial relationships between commercial sponsors and CME providers" (2009). Commercial sponsors' main focus is profitability for their stock holders. This causes a conflict of interest in our medical community. Our health care system needs proven results, not a reliance on a broken system which drains resources for the profits of big corporations.

Chapter 4
Particulars about Different Groups

Social-emotional Behavior and Cognitive Development of Children

Have you ever noticed that we all start our lives with rhythm? The first thing we are ever aware of in our mother's womb is the steady rhythmic beating of our mother's heart. We become entrained to that rhythm. After birth, our mothers instinctively rock us; the steady rhythm lulls us. "Mothers around the world sing lullabies to their babies, and research findings suggest the benefit can be dramatic, particularly for infants born prematurely" (Dossey, p. 98, 2006). Our first learning experiences are through rhythmic exercises such as learning the ABC song. Cognitively underdeveloped children, such as those with autism, instinctively rock to their own rhythm. None of this is coincidence; scientists have proven that we are rhythmic beings down to the quantum level.

When working with social-emotional behavior and cognitive development with children, RMT can be used effectively. Drumming and meditation have been shown to enhance prosocial behavior (Kokal, et al., 2011). "School counselor-led group drumming, integrated with activities from group counseling, appears to improve the social and emotional correlates of chronic stress in low-income children. Through a positive development approach, the program can increase core assets that may influence a wide spectrum of behaviors, thus yielding broad public health value" (Ho, Tsao, Bloch, & Zelter, 2010). This research shows a direct correlation between stress and stress related diseases and drumming through controlled experiments with low-income children in actual school settings. Children who were in the drumming group showed significant reduction in stress related symptoms and gained greater control over adverse behavioral problems. "Music sooths the savage beast" (William Congreve). This research has a direct relation to my larger subject due to evidence of stress relief and decrease in stress related symptoms used in a realistic school environment. It also shows that the drumming is only part of the behavioral change, but also includes the inclusion in a group event. Social inclusion (peer pressure) is a powerful tool in modifying behavior. The children showed changes in ADHD, inattentiveness, opposition defiant problems, PTSD, and sluggish cognitive development. (Ho, et al., 2010). The earlier we can start children in these types of programs, the more tools they will have to adapt to their environment in the future, and the less likely they are to develop greater problems along the way.

In an article by Kimberly Sena Moore in Psychology Today, she shows empirical evidence for drumming, in helping children with social, emotional, motor, and cognitive development (2011). She lists these things for children with special needs, and says that drumming can be a powerful tool to help them address:

- **Social Needs**. Drumming often occurs as a collaborative, interactive process. If facilitated correctly, participating in drumming experiences can help a child work on skills such as turn-taking and sharing, as well as help them feel they are part of a group contributing towards a group process.
- **Communication Needs**. Playing a drum or percussion instrument can be a useful way to communicate nonverbally and to "listen" to another person's nonverbal communication.
- **Fine and Gross Motor Skills**. This may almost seem self-evident, but different playing techniques can be used to help work on different fine and gross motor skills. This can even be true for developing lower extremity strength (e.g. imagine standing and playing a large conga drum).
- **Emotional Needs**. Participating in a drumming activity can help a child feel safe enough to express his/her feelings. Additionally--and speaking from experience--there's nothing much better for releasing anger than banging on a drum.
- **Cognitive Needs**. By participating in a drumming experience, children can be working on attention, impulse control, and decision-making skills.

Each one of these points hits core basics for a child's development and also increases true self-esteem.

Our self-esteem is at the root of who we are, how we perceive ourselves in society, and who we become. True self-esteem comes from internal sources such as self-responsibility, self-sufficiency, and the knowledge of one's own competence and capability to deal with obstacles and adversities, and the security of knowing where we fit in our world. For too many years we have been using a method which involves judging and then reflecting. Studies over the past 30 years have focused on this false method of self-esteem and shown that this doesn't work and therefore the issue has been invalidated. Most people today deal with self-esteem issues and will struggle with it to their grave. If we deal with self-esteem issues while the child is in their formative years, we may be able to change the paths of the next Columbine.

From the time we are conceived to the time we die, rhythm plays a vital role in how we develop. Since the beginning of recorded history, rhythm has been discussed for development and healing. In Larry Dossey's book *The Extraordinary Healing Power of Ordinary Things*, he talks about how both Plato and Socrates agreed that rhythm is vital to education of children (p. 94, 2006). He goes on to point out how religions and governments down through history have tried to control music because of the power that rhythm has upon our bodies and minds (p. 95-97, 2006). Why are we not using rhythm from the moment of birth and through our children's formative years to enhance their chances of succeeding? Yet, it is the first program to be pulled in schools when funding gets short. Think about it; governments want control. You can't control people who are educated enough to know you are controlling them.

Drugs and Alcohol

Drum circles for drug and alcohol recovery have been shown to effect "physiological dynamics, inducing the relaxation response and restoring balance in the opioid and serotonergic neurotransmitter systems. Psychodynamic needs for self-awareness and insight, emotional healing, and psychological integration. Spiritual needs for contact with a higher power and spiritual experiences. Social needs for connectedness with others and interpersonal support" (Winkelman, 2003). Whether it is the need to express ourselves emotionally or be shown a group activity where people can enjoy themselves without the use of drugs or alcohol, drumming can get you there. Again, the only drawback is getting people past their fear of making mistakes or being ridiculed for participating. 'The physiological effects of drumming and the positive effects of group drumming experiences on recovery that are attested to by counselors who have incorporated these activities into substance abuse rehabilitation programs provide a compelling rationale for the utilization and evaluation of this resource" (Winkelman, 2003).

Stress increases the chance of "relapsing in to drug use" (Sapolsky, p.349, 2004). "One of the important predictors for successful completion of recovery from addictions is *self-efficacy*, or the degree of confidence that the addict has what it takes to stay clean and sober" (Phillips, p.60, 2000). Starting with something as simple as drumming, individuals can step right into being a creative functioning part of a supportive group. Each person can be proud of what they contribute, no matter how small or how large within the music. This increases self esteem and confidence.

Dementia /Alzheimer's/Parkinson's

Dementia and Alzheimer's disease clients will only be able to do RMT in their early stages. Mid or late stage dementia and Parkinson's disease needs a different approach. They can still get benefits from the rhythm, but due to physical and mental deterioration, just sitting and listening or participating with some type of percussion instrument may be all they can do in later stages. What I have found in my own work with dementia patients is that they may not recognize me each session, but they do react to the rhythm quicker and quicker each time, each in their own way at their own pace. During my internship in a severe dementia ward, I worked with a lady who could become verbally abusive very quickly. She was the first resident that was pointed out to me by the staff. The first day I came and played my drum there, she got up right away cursing and walked out. Each time I came, she progressively stayed longer and when she did go out, she sat nearer and nearer to the room. I even caught her a couple of times vocalizing with a beat between times the group was playing together. Finally she stayed in the room through one whole session and actually played a shaker and smiled during her playing. The next time I came, she again walked out right away and sat in the adjoining room. I was not thrown off thinking something was wrong; I have been teaching drums long enough to see unimpaired students do the same thing. It is a natural cycle of progression and regression, then progressing again to a higher level.

Alzheimer's is a degenerative disease that can affect memory, language, and judgment (Sacks, p. 336, 2007). "People with severe Alzheimer's cannot communicate and are completely dependent on others for their care. Near the end, the person may be in bed most or all of the time as the body shuts down" (Alzheimer's disease, 2011). This puts daily increasing burdens on the care giving staff.

Oliver Sacks, in his book *Musicophilia,* tells us that "music perception, music sensibility, music emotion, and music memory can survive long after other forms of memory have disappeared" (p. 337, 2007). Music therapy "seeks to address the emotions, cognitive powers, thoughts, and memories, the surviving 'self' of the patient, to stimulate these and bring them to the fore. It aims to enrich and enlarge existence, to give freedom, stability, organization and focus" (Sacks, p. 336-337, 2007). Dementia can come from various causes "…from multiple strokes, from cerebral hypoxia, from toxic or metabolic abnormalities, from brain injuries or infections, from frontotemporal degeneration or most commonly from Alzheimer's disease" (Sacks, p. 335, 2007).

So far, there is no cure for dementia or Alzheimer's disease. The only thing that can be done is to watch the progression and give as much comfort to the patient as possible as they deteriorate. This brings me to another point regarding dementia and Alzheimer's; the health and mental wellness of end-of-life care-givers. Compassion fatigue (or secondary traumatic stress) has emerged as a natural consequence of caring for clients who are in pain, suffering or traumatized" (Compassion fatigue and nursing work: can we accurately capture the consequences of caring work? 2006).

Compassion Fatigue

Through my own experiences and from my research, I have found caregivers for dementia and Alzheimer's patients seem to struggle more than any other types of care givers, although it is not easy for any caregiver. Assisting someone that you know will never recover and takes more and more care each day as the disease progresses, takes a severe toll on the physical, mental and emotional wellbeing of the caregivers. This increases their vulnerability to stress related disease. "Little emphasis has been placed on the potential health consequences for nurses providing care and caring within the health-care system. Compassion fatigue (or secondary traumatic stress) has emerged as a natural consequence of caring for clients who are in pain, suffering or traumatized"

(Compassion fatigue and nursing work: can we accurately capture the consequences of caring work? 2006).

RMT can be an excellent release for compassion fatigue. By helping the caregivers relieve their stress, it will help the overall environment of the situation and carry back over to the patient. The question is, can any facility afford not to support reversing stress and stress related issues in the work place before they become an issue? They could cost the company in things such as in/out patient visits on insurance or over all loses of productivity and more. I have found over the years that attitude-enhancing changes in a work place can mean the difference between making and breaking a company. As healthcare costs go up, competent employees are going to be harder to keep; each facility running on bare budgets. A little money spent on them now will help motivate employees and make a better working environment which will be sustainable over the long run.

PTSD

Post-Traumatic Stress Disorder (PTSD) is the name of a condition for someone who has had a traumatic experience with symptoms that last longer than six months (Naparstek, p. 35, 2006).

> "Trauma memories are not absorbed by the thinking brain, the way ordinary memories are. Rather they are shelved in disconnected sensory fragments, somatic sensations, and muscular impulses, in the more

primitive areas of the brain. As such, they are walled off, disconnected from awareness, and inaccessible to cognition. Nor do they fade over time; instead, they either maintain their original strength or grow even more intense, fueled by repetition" (Naparstek, p. 27, 2006). "We now understand that an individual's history of psychiatric problems increases the odds of PTSD, as do lower education, subsequent stress, and lack of social support" (Naparstek, p.67, 2006).

PTSD is not just a soldier's disease. Anyone who has been in stressful situations for long periods of time or exposed to trauma can get PTSD. This can include children who have been abused or bullied, people who have been involved in violent crimes such as rape or spousal abuse (both mental and physical), anyone who has been part of or witnessed traumatic events (first responders), ongoing cancer victims, just to name a few. This could also include someone who has chronic anxiety or has lost a loved one. On a web site put out by The National Institute of Mental Health on PTSD, it states that 7.7 million Americans are affected by PTSD. This is a staggering number, and there are probably many more that go undiagnosed. Again, the key word in all this is stress. Anything that will help with stress factors is going to help with PTSD. The parasympathetic system is crucial in reversing the damage done. But again, if the sympathetic system has been going non-stop, that becomes the operant conditioning. The body will not understand what relax means and will therefore reject the parasympathetic system as something foreign. The body will have to be retrained to make relaxation be the new operant conditioning. RMT can do this in a natural and nonintrusive way.

Soldiers

The stigma of mental health treatment in the military operates from the stereotype that soldiers who seek treatment are weak. Perceptions of weakness derive from the belief that treatment violates military norms of group cohesion and individualistic coping. The cognitive dissonance created by the fear and by the stigma creates a barrier to any form of real healing or empowerment of the individual. In a study done by Dias, Oda, Akiba, Arruda, and Bruder (2009) cognitive dissonance impaired performance of tasks "regardless of rewards, punishments and any method to produce motivational contradictions" (p. 788). This means impaired judgment for individuals wishing to make informed decisions about their lives. This cognitive dissonance tends to make individuals withdraw within themselves rather than facing those fears. By not facing these fears, further damage is caused to the psyche.

The best way to fight cognitive dissonance is through information and understanding of the problem. "Research on the action-based model suggests that dissonance reduction may serve the function of assisting in the successful execution of a commitment, which may facilitate effective and unconflicted action" (Harmon-Jones & Harmon-Jones, 2007, p. 13). Empowerment of each individual is the basis for permanent change within ourselves and our communities.

RMT can work for any type of PTSD; soldiers can use the drum to help with some of their particular circumstances such as hyper-vigilance with loud noises. During my internship at the VA Medical Center in Lakewood, Washington, there was one veteran who would only come in and stay for about five minutes, but would just beat on the drum as hard as he could; not even staying with the rhythm everyone else was setting. He would then get up, rubbing his hands, and walk out. After a couple of times of this I was growing concerned that he might be affecting the other participants and I brought it up to the group. They assured me that they were all just fine with it and told me that normally he could be very abrasive to everyone, but after the days he participated, he was much calmer and easier to get along with. He just needed a safe way of releasing his tensions, anxieties and frustrations. I thought back to my first drumming experiences and remembered having people tell me to lighten up on my hitting of the drum. Later, my African teacher told me to disregard those comments and do what I felt that I needed to do; the subtleties would come later once I worked through what I needed to work through. Frustration and anger need a safe outlet. Regular RMT can facilitate self-expression and provide a channel for transforming frustration, anger, and aggression into the experience of creativity and self-mastery.

The operant conditioning which results from gunfire or explosions can be difficult for standard therapies. By starting out soft and rhythmic with the drumming, the therapist can change that operant conditioning of sounds into a non-threatening and empowering experience for the client. In the book *The Healing Power of Drums* by Robert Friedman, he tells about a group of Vietnam veterans that by the end of their program were creating the sounds of battles with their drums. "This was the thing that they were most scared of, and they were in control of it. They were making these sounds of battle, and no one was getting hurt" (Freidman, p.110, 2000). This also reinforces the point that feeling in control of our environment helps to relieve the effects of stress.

Team Building

To be a successful company, you have to build powerful and cohesive teams which are focused on the group company agenda rather than an individual agenda. This means having people who know how to work as a team. This type of program does not use the whole RMT method. Rather, it uses more of a facilitated drum circle model and involves debriefing and discussion to highlight key points and helps relate the experience back to the workplace.

Musicians have always known about the strong bonds of being in a performance group together, but for the average person this is a new and extraordinarily powerful experience with many benefits to the individual and a company workforce. To make any kind of music, the group has to be able to work together. Drumming takes no prior talent to achieve that end. It just takes listening, feeling the rhythm, and cooperating with the dominant beat of your fellow participants. I hear all the time, "I can't participate because I have no rhythm." Yet, those same people have a heart that beats at a steady rhythm, walk at a steady rhythm, or even tap on their steering wheel to the beat of their favorite song. We can't stop ourselves from participating in the rhythm of songs in some way. Every molecule in our body vibrates to a regular rhythm. Drumming takes advantage of that natural entrainment. From the story I told earlier about the 90 year old gentleman who didn't think he was adding anything to the group; he demonstrated the value of an individual's contribution to the group at whatever level they are comfortable with. Drumming unites different personality types and embraces diversity. Because there is no right or wrong way to participate in the steady rhythm, it lowers stress, helps focus the mind, allows for improvisation and creativity, promotes cooperation and effective non-verbal communication, and also encourages positive risk taking. Through rhythm games, drumming can instill leadership skills and shared leadership dynamics while energizing and uplifting any group.

Chapter 5

Healthcare Costs

The current healthcare costs in this country are non-sustainable. "The cost of insurance premiums and employee medical claims is at an all time high and continues to rise. Business leaders are being called upon to make changes at the workplace in order to curb rising costs. Many are turning to workplace health programs to help employees adopt healthier lifestyles and lower their risk of developing costly chronic diseases" (CDC, 2011)

Many of the methods discussed in this book have been shown, that each of these independent modalities can do more than just stabilize the person, but actually reverse the damage done by stress and trauma. By reversing the damage done, the body can go back to regulating itself with little to no pharmacological or psychological help. Often there are PTSD survivors that thrive from their use. "Getting in touch with these powerful human capabilities and spiritual connections that have popped open from the adrenergized terror state leads to more joy, more aliveness, and more productivity in the months and years to come" (Naparstek, p. 94, 2006). This saves costs and takes the strain off of our healthcare system. RMT can decrease the amount of psychotherapy, decrease emergency visits, decrease the amount of medication needed, decrease in and out patient visits, and increase productivity in the work place, all through stress reduction alone. Since stress seems to be the common factor, let stress relieving methods lead the way. As Mahatma Gandhi once said "Be the change you want to see in the world."

Chapter 6

Social Change through Sound Community Psychology

Real changes in our healthcare community cannot be done by individuals. It takes a community to bind together to create real social change. The field of Community Psychology gives us proven methods to look at, support, and make real, lasting changes in our communities. "Community psychology (CP) is an action-orientated field that strives to address problems and create change" (Nelson & Prilleltensky, 2010, p. 1). CP is about working alongside disadvantaged people to bring about inspiration and better uses of resources for the greater good of the whole community. Community psychologists look at problems from the micro, meso, and macro levels and apply core values and principles to come up with solutions which create ameliorative and transformative changes within communities. The values of CP are based more on "what should be, not what is" (Nelson & Prilleltensky, 2010, p. 34) because of structural and historical problems which have been deeply rooted in past social reconstruction. These values include such things as holism, health, caring and compassion, self-determination, diversity, and accountability (Nelson & Prilleltensky, 2010, p. 35). The key principles used by CP are applied at the personal, relational and collective levels to the greater good of all within the community. They include ecology, prevention and promotion, community, power, inclusion, commitment, and empowerment (Nelson & Prilleltensky, 2010, p. 35). This form of intervention does not allow for greed or self promotion. It is about doing the most good for the greatest number.

Because of CP's scientific basis, it sets itself apart from community based action groups and social and political movements (Nelson & Prilleltensky 2010, p. 41). This is to minimize the tendency to convert back to the status quo (Nelson & Prilleltensky 2010, p. 43). No matter whether it is intentional or not, we as a society get stuck into this status quo and find ways of justifying or rationalizing our position. CP is about making real and lasting changes within our communities for the betterment of the whole community.

In Maton's (2008) article on empowerment within the community he writes, "…the empowering change process encompasses transformations in group-based belief system, core educational activities, relational environment, and opportunity role structure" (p. 16).

Bringing people closer together in thought and action is a greater part of Community Psychology. We all need to look at where we are and what is going on with others around us. By looking and acting as individuals, we get individual results, but lose our identity within the larger group. By acting as a group/community, we make gains within the collective and also define ourselves.

I have written this book as a way of showing that there are viable, cheaper, sustainable options to the status quo which is currently not working. It is about raising a voice to say there is a better way.

Chapter 7
Summary

After I started drumming back in the late 1990's, I went in for my regular check up and my doctor told me I was progressing well and asked me what I had been taking to help fight my stress and depression. I told him I was drumming. He laughed and asked, "No really, what are you taking?" Again, I told him I was just drumming. He told me that drumming wouldn't make the change he was seeing in me. That is the same form of thought that I have encountered from many in the medical field. I have even been told that my "airy fairy new age crap is not real" by a doctor, because he knew more than I did; he had a degree in medicine. Don't get me wrong, not everyone in the medical field thinks that way, but I have had some resistance to alternate forms of thought due to the status quo. At the beginning of my class in mind-body medicine, one of our faculty quoted Albert Einstein when he said, "We can't solve problems by using the same kind of thinking we used when we created them." This is the motivation for my research and this new form of therapy. We can't do the same things over and over again and expect different results. Quantum physics tells us we are just vibrating particles. Wouldn't that make you think that a vibrational medicine should be at the basis of all health modalities? It could be used for preventative medicine as well as recovery. Many people in the medical field are now able to see the results being found due to new tests and brain imaging devices. This new brain imaging is bringing up all kinds of new research fields into sounds' and thoughts' effects upon the biological systems of the body.

In this book I have shown that this form of healing modality can change us down to our genetic level. Modern Western Medicine has not been able to show the same results. "The vast majority of pharmaceutical drugs do not heal disease—they control symptoms by introducing chemical mediators, at specific levels, into the body" (Buhner, p. 84, 2002). Dr. Mehl-Madrona echoes that same thought when he said, "we actually do not have evidence to support the universal superiority of pharmaceuticals over all other forms of therapy" (p. 93, 2007). He goes on to say, "Researchers at Beth Israel Deaconess Medical Center and Harvard Medical School finally did such a study and found that a nondrug approach—cognitive-behavioral therapy—was better than drugs" (p. 93, 2007). Mental health counselors are finding the same things with their old way of thinking with talk therapy. "If a deeply traumatized person is prompted *only* to speak and think about the event that created his distress, without enlisting help from the imaginal, emotional, sensory, and somatic capabilities of his right brain, his symptoms can actually get worse instead of better" (Naparstek, p.XVIII, 2006). This is not to say that there is not also a place for Western medicine. It is excellent at emergency and stabilization techniques and I respect it for that, but once the person is stabilized, then the healing should begin. We need to step around our old biases and look at facts. Drumming and meditation heal the body and the mind. By combining the two together, we can work towards a healthier society and bring down the costs of our unsustainable healthcare system. It allows us to be able to vent our emotions in a safe and artistic way. It allows us to communicate at a much deeper level without getting out of our own comfort level; each adding what they can, when they can, at whatever level they can, in an environment without right or wrong: only acceptance and expression of yourself. It doesn't matter whether you are a first time beginner or an experienced drummer, each is adding their voice to the community song; one as needed as the other.

    The first thing we are ever aware of from the time of our conception on this planet is the rhythm of our cells dividing and the rhythm of our mother's heart and body around us. Rhythm goes to the base of who we are. Anywhere I have ever played, people of all ages start to dance or tap to the rhythm of the drums. It brings out a whole body reaction in the listener as well as the players. A child that can barely stand, holding on to his stroller, bopping to the music in the park, teens in schools creating their own rhythms, Buddhist Nuns dancing in a monastery dining room, or the severely demented elderly lady at the nursing home kicking her arms and legs to the beat of the drums because it is the only way she has left to express herself; we all feel it. It comes from a deeper part of us that still seems to be there when time, disease, and injury have taken everything else away. Shouldn't that be where we are starting our healing from?

Appendix

A Brief Overview of RMT

RMT starts with a group which is verbally guided through a mindfulness meditation which lasts from 20 to 30 minutes. Then, the clients are led through a series of expressive drumming experiences to close out the hour to hour and a half session. I prefer the West African Djembe drum because of its ability to cover a wide variety of sounds and because it can be played with both hands, although any hand drum will work. On the surface this may sound simple, but like any healing modality, there is much more behind the scene. It is about targeting specific neural functions to elicit neural growth. This is what a normal session would look like.

At first invite the clients to sit down. An invitation is much less obtrusive and helps set the tone for what is to come. Have a drum put out in front of each chair. Don't mention the drum; drumming is "too hard" is the main reaction you'll get, so don't use the term drumming. Sitting next to it, they are meeting the drum half way. Begin by having them start breathing and paying attention to that breathing. We have become a society of shallow breathers. Without enough oxygen in the system, the system can't work at optimum efficiency. Therefore, throughout the whole session, it is good at regular intervals to *remind* the participants to pay attention to their breathing. Every type of meditation that I have encountered starts with the breath. As you are getting them to focus on the breath, start tapping on the edge of the drum. Nothing complicated, just a slow, steady, right-left-right-left. "If anything, it's best to focus on the kinesthetic or feeling senses as the premier perceptional avenue for healing" (Naparstek, p. 203, 2006). The drum is a hands-on experience that draws you in. "Music plays a powerful and underappreciated role in increasing the power of guided imagery, and just as with the voice, effective music does not draw attention to itself or compete with the listener's images by being too interesting in and of itself" (Naparstek, p. 193, 2006).

Ask the clients to go ahead and close their eyes once they see what you are doing and have them settled and breathing. Don't worry about asking them to hit the drum; they will be drawn to start tapping along with the beat you set. One purpose of both hands tapping is because the tapping causes bilateral stimulation across both hemispheres in the brain. This is like exercising the connection (corpus callosum) between the right and left hemispheres in the brain for a "whole brain" approach much like EMDR (Eye Movement Desensitization and Reprocessing) (Phillips, p. 9, 2000). It is very relaxing and calming.

Keep your voice soft and even as you slowly start having them pay attention to the different parts of their bodies. Voice quality and intonation can make the difference between a good session and a bad one. "Your voice is there to provide a quiet, trustworthy, undistracting platform from which the listener can access his or her unique reactions and responses. So your voice can't be calling attention to itself. Neither should there be even hints of seduction, manipulative, or controlling flavor" (Naparstek, p. 193, 2006). I start at the mouth because of the breathing and work from there through each sense in the head, asking them to experience that part of themselves here and now, and then start working down through the body taking the time to experience each part from the point of view of each sense, audibly, visually, or kinetically. Spend a little time on each part of the body, having them notice feelings and sensations in each part (Naparstek, p. 168, 2006). "As simple as this sequence is, it can have a profound effect on a disembodied, disconnected person, offering a physical feeling of stability and a relaxed groundedness they didn't even know was missing" (Naparstek, p. 168, 2006). By the time I get through to the shoulders, I ask them if they could get 5 percent more comfortable, to go ahead and do it then. I then return to the breathing again by having them start feeling their chest rise and fall with the breath. Once they have settled, return to slowly working down through the body, paying attention to each part, repeating your chosen operant wording. I use "here and now." This is a form of operant conditioning which, with each session they do, will train the mind to think in the here and now; becoming easier and easier each time to stay in the here and now. The right-left tapping on the drum will help this physically anchor on the subconscious level. As this goes along, they may have a tendency to speed up the tapping. If you can't control it through entrainment, verbally slow them down to keep a slow steady pace. Entrainment is defined as "the tendency of people and objects to synchronize to a dominant rhythm" (Friedman, p.43, 2000). This practice will bring all the body into the here and now, not just the mind. Once you have worked through the whole body from end to end, allow the people to keep tapping and pay attention to the thoughts that may come into their minds without judgment and just look at each thought as it comes. Let them experience that for a short time before moving on. Pay attention to the nonverbal clues the group gives for the length of any exercise.

At this point ask them to pick one short term goal they would like to achieve. Have them phrase it and see it in their mind as if it is happening now. Have them go through each sense. What would it look like? Would there be any smells? Would you taste anything? What would you hear? After each one, leave a pause so they have time to experience what might come into their minds. This allows all the senses to connect fully with the image (Phillips, p. 107, 2000). Since our focus determines our reality, by visualizing our goal in greater detail, we have a better frame of reference to start creating it. In the book *Finding the Energy to Heal*, Maggie Phillips makes the statement, "Although imagery is not thought of as an energy therapy approach, it is a basic staple of human experience, and therefore of any treatment" (p. 231, 2000). She also goes on to state, "…the healing effects of imagery with mindbody health symptoms are perhaps more widely documented than any other healing methods" (p. 231, 2000). "Don't worry if the imagery brings forth unexpected emotions. It has a way of making people tearful, either because their hearts are touched, or because they are releasing grief, or both" (Naparstek, p. 203, 2006). You also have the option of other visual imagery at this time depending on the needs of the group. "Many people with health issues benefit from images on experiences of past mastery in order to prepare for future challenges" (Phillips, p. 117, 2000).

I end this portion of the session by having them imagine a bright, healing white energy coming up through their feet and slowly enveloping their entire body. As they feel the energy slowly rise, I instruct them to slowly open their eyes and return to the room and I also slowly increase the speed of the tapping on the drum until it turns into a rumble; I then stop. Allow the room to be quiet for a few minutes and let them process the experience before starting anything else. This powerful ending can have a very dramatic effect. You may have people who will need to share afterwards. It is about allowing without dominance.

Experiential Drumming

This part of the program is designed to allow each participant to explore their own inner rhythms within the larger group. It is meant to allow them to feel empowered. Don't try to teach any rhythms, that put pressure on the participants and doesn't allow them to share freely and will cause more stress. In a research paper titled Synchronized drumming enhances activity in the caudate and facilitates prosocial commitment - if the rhythm comes, it says that if the participants aren't worried whether they are doing it right or wrong, drumming can precipitate more activity in the caudate region of the brain, "a region associated with reward processing" (Kokal, Engel, Kirschner, & Keysers, 2011), thereby increasing a better chance of health rewards. I have had participants sing, tone, or just vocalize during this part of the session. Because this is about letting go and letting out our inner selves, this can be very helpful. Don't be afraid to join in or just encourage them with non-verbal communication. Remind them to breathe before, during, and after each rhythm.

    I like to start with an easy rhythm with a strong, steady down beat. The steadiness of the down beat is critical, don't vary it. It is a good metaphor for our whole lives. The one thing that all of us seem to look for in our lives is consistency. It has been shown in psychology that any phase of our lives can be disrupted without consistency. This goes back to what I talked about earlier from Sapolsky's book when he stated that predictability is fundamental to decreasing stress (p.258, 2004). This is important for all the rhythms you play with the group. You can vary within the rhythm, but don't vary the base rhythm. I don't let any rhythm go more than five to seven minutes usually, because of our short human attention spans. That is longer than most songs we hear on the radio; but that is a judgment call by the facilitator. Pay attention to the group. Because of entrainment, I usually start fading out quietly and everyone else follows. If they keep going, let them go until it comes to a group conclusion.

The next rhythm I use is a heartbeat rhythm with a long break in it. I have everyone just listen for a short time before they start playing and just verbally repeat after me. Base-base-tap-tap-tap-tap-base-base (big pause) base-base-tap-tap-tap-tap-base-base (big pause). Keep repeating this rhythm and say the "big pause" for the first few times they go through it. Due to entrainment, they will join in with the rhythm and leave the space in. This verbalization also helps with the rhythm. I have had several teachers tell me that if you can say it, you can play it. The association between the thought and the action anchors the rhythm in the mind. After a couple of minutes, encourage them to add something simple into the pause space and then let someone else do it the next time around. This allows some to get their own voices heard within the rhythm. Tell them it is much like a conversation, not everyone can talk at once; take turns. You may have to give them an example to follow, such as an extra "tap-tap" in the space to get them started, then back out and let them go. As before, pay attention to the group and allow it to come to its best conclusion. Again, don't try to teach them the rhythm. Some may do it exactly like you do, and some won't; allow that to be all right. This is about encouraging them to open themselves more within the group. There is no right or wrong.

Another good rhythm game to play which can be very useful is to pick a good affirmation that is appropriate for the group you are working with and let them try to put a rhythm to it. Try something like "I am worthy and deserving—yes I am." Say the phrase several times in a sing-song way, and then show them how to follow the sing-song with a rhythm on the drums. After you have tried one, ask the group if there is one they would like to try. This allows the group to have some control over the music being played. Control is one of the features listed by Sapolsky as essential for stress reduction (p. 260-263, 2004). Repetition of the affirmation helps anchor the phrase into their subconscious. "When we concentrate attention repeatedly on a goal or idea, it tends to be realized" (Hammond, p.12, 1990). I have found that this exercise can quite often end in laughter; laughter is a great medicine in itself.

The rest of the time, I start playing with a base rhythm and get more and more advanced within the base rhythm. This encourages the participants to start exploring within the rhythm. Don't allow yourself to get too loud and overpower the group. This is about showing them that they can get outside of the base rhythm and explore and not to show off what you can do. It is very important to smile and make eye contact with each individual within the group during the exploration part of the session. Be sure to nod and give encouragement throughout. Body language is very important in a drum session. The facilitator will be the one everyone will be looking to for approval and acceptance. This will set the tone for the whole group. Your demeanor throughout will be watched by the group. The more confidence and enjoyment you show, the more effective the session will be.

The beating on the drums throughout the whole session allows for a physical and emotional release of stress and energy, and best of all, has no known side effects. What better way can there be to work off frustrations, anger, and aggression in a creative and non-violent way?

There are a myriad of other percussion and drumming games that can be used for targeting specific outcomes. Don't be afraid to look and try new things. New things create more neural growth and fight repetition and boredom.

Contact Information

www.Outlawdrummers.com

Bill@outlawdrummers.com

REFERENCES

Baeck, E. (2002). The neural networks of music. *European Journal of Neurology, 9,* 449-456.

Bandler, R., & Grinder, J. (1975). *Patterns of the hypnotic techniques of Milton H. Erickson, M.D.* (Vol. 1). Capitola, CA: Meta.

Bieszczad, K. M., & Weinberger, N. M. (2012). Extinction reveals that primary sensory cortex predicts reinforcement outcome. *European Journal of Neuroscience, 35,* 598-613. http://dx.doi.org/10.1111/j.1460-9568.2011.07974.x

Bittman, B., Berk, L. S., Felten, D. L., Westengard, J., Simonton, O. C., Pappas, J., & Ninehouser, M. (2001). Composite effects of group drumming music therapy on modulation of neuroendocrine-immune parameters in normal subjects. Alternative Therapies, 7.

Bittman, B., Berk, L., Shannon, M., Sharaf, M., Westengard, J., Guegler, K. J., & Ruff, D. W. (2005). Recreational music-making modulates the human stress response: a preliminary individualized gene expression strategy. *Med Sci Monit, 11*(2).

Blackburn, E. H., Greider, C. W., & Szostak, J. W. (2006). Telomeres and telomerase: The path from maize, Tetrahymena and yeast to human cancer and aging. *Nature Medicine, 12*(10).

Buhner, S. H. (2002). *The lost language of plants.* White Rivers Junction, VT:

Chelsea Green.

Compassion fatigue and nursing work: can we accurately capture the consequences of caring work? (2006). In US national library of medicine national institutes of health. Retrieved from US National Library of Medicine National Institutes of Health database.

Cook, M. (2004). *Who can cure the pharmaceuticals?*. *New Statesman, 133(4714)*, 29-30.

Crane, B. (1998). *Reflexology: A basic guide*. New York, NY: Barnes & Noble.

Dias, Á., Oda, E., Akiba, H., Arruda, L., & Bruder, L. (2009). Is Cognitive Dissonance an Intrinsic Property of the Human Mind? An Experimental Solution to a Half-Century Debate. World Academy Of Science, Engineering & Technology, 54784-788.

Doidge, N. (2007). *The brain that changes itself*. New York, NY: Penguin Group.

Dossey, L. (2006). *The extraordinary healing power of ordinary things: Fourteen natural steps to health and happiness*. New York, NY: Harmony Books.

Epel, E., Daubenmier, J., Moskowitz, J. T., Folkman, S., & Blackburn, E. (2009, August). *Can meditation slow rate of cellular aging? Cognitive stress mindfulness, and telomeres,* San Francisco, CA: Ann N Y Acad Sci.

Friedman, R. L. (2000). *The healing power of the drum*. Reno, NV: White Cliff Media.

Hammond, D. C. (Ed.). (1990). Handbook of hypnotic suggestions and metaphors. New York, NY: W. W. Norton & Company.

Hanh, T. N. (2009). Answers from the heart: Practical responses to life's burning questions. Berkeley, CA: Parallax Press.

Harmon-Jones, E., & Harmon-Jones, C. (2007). Cognitive dissonance theory after 50 years of development. Zeitschrift für Sozialpsychologie, 38(1), 13.

Harrington, A. (2008). The cure within: A history of mind-body medicine. New York: W.W. Norton.

Ho, P., Tsao, J. C.I., Bloch, L., & Zelter, L. K. (2010). The impact of group drumming on social-emotional. Evidence-Based Complementary and Alternative Medicine, 2011. doi:10.1093/ecam/neq072

Horowitz, S. (2004). *Evidence-based reflexology. Alternative & Complementary Therapies.*

Huang, T. L., & Charyton, C. (2008). A comprehensive review of the psychological effects of *brainwave entrainment* [Fact sheet]. Retrieved January 29, 2013, from US National Library of Medicine website: http://www.ncbi.nlm.nih.gov/pubmed/18780583

Kannathal, N., Paul, J. K., Lim, C. M., & Chua, K. P. (2004). Effect of reflexology on eeg – A nonlinear approach. *The American Journal of Chinese Medicine, 32*(4), 641-650.

Kasprzak, C. (2011). Influence of binaural beats on EEG signal. Acta Physica Polonica A: Acoustic and Biomedical Engineering, 119.

Kokal, I., Engel, A., Kirschner, S., & Keysers, C. (2011). Synchronized drumming enhances activity in the caudate and facilitates prosocial commitment - if the rhythm comes easily. Bologna, Italy: PLoS ONE. doi:10.1371/journal.pone.0027272

Lane, J. D., Kasian, S. J., Owens, J. E., & Marsh, G. R. (1998). Binaural auditory beats affect vigilance performance and mood. *Physiology & Behavior*, *63*(2), 249-252.

Maton, K. I. (2008). Empowering community settings: Agents of individual development, community betterment, and positive social change [Data file]. University of Maryland, MD: Department of psychology.

Mehl-Madrona, L. (2007). Narrative medicine: the use of history and story in the healing process. Rochester, VT: Bear & Co.

Moore, K. S. (2011, March 10). Drumming for development: how drumming helps children with special needs. *Psychology Today*.

Naparstek, B. (2006). *Invisible heroes: Survivors of trauma and how they heal*. New York, NY: Bantam Dell.

Nelson, G., & Prilleltensky, I. (2010). Community psychology: In pursuit of liberation and well-being (2nd ed.). New York, NY: Palgrave Macmillian.

Office of inspector general Department of health and human services. (2009, July). *Commercial sponsorship of continuing medical education* (L. Morris, Comp.).

Phillips, M. (2000). Finding the energy to heal: How EMDR, hypnosis, TFT, imagery, and body-focused therapy can help restore mindbody health. New York, NY: W.W. Norton & Company.*Post-traumatic stress disorder* [Fact sheet]. (n.d.). Retrieved September 25, 2013, from The National Institute of Mental Health website: http://www.nimh.nih.gov/health/topics/post-traumatic-stress-disorder-ptsd/index.shtml

Post-Traumatic Stress Disorder: Evidence-based research for the third millennium [Review of the literature [Title of Reviewed Work], performed by J. Iribarren, P. Prolo, N. Neagos, & F. Chiappelli]. (2005). *Oxford University Press*, 503-512. http://dx.doi.org/10.1093/ecam/neh127

Rising health care costs are unsustainable. (2011, April 25). Retrieved from Centers for Disease Control and Prevention website:http://www.cdc.gov/workplacehealthpromotion/businesscase/reasons/rising.html

Sacks, O. (2007). Musicophilia. Alfred A. Knopf.

Sapolsky, R. M. (2004). *Why zebras don't get ulcers*. New York, NY: Henry Holt and Company.

Stevens, C. (2012). *Music medicine*. Boulder, CO: Sounds True.

Stress. (2012). In *Oxford dictionary*. Retrieved from http://oxforddictionaries.com/definition/ English/stress.

The Tucker Foundation and Dartmouth Hitchcock Medical Center. (2011, April

13). *Jon Kabat*-Zinn - "The healing power of mindfulness" [Video file]. Retrieved from http://www.youtube.com/watch?v=_If4a-gHg_I

U.S. Department of Health and Human Services National Institutes of Health. (2011, July). *Alzheimer's disease* (Report No. 11-6423).

Vujanovic, Niles, Pietrefesa, Potter, & Schmertz. (2011). Potential of mindfulness in treating trauma reactions. Retrieved July 23, 2013, from Department of Veterans Affairs website: http://www.ptsd.va.gov/professional/pages/mindful-PTSD.asp

Wahbeh, H., Calabrese, C., & Zwickey, H. (2007). Binaural beat technology in humans: A pilot study to assess psychologic and physiologic effects. *The Journal of Alternative and Complementary Medicine, 13*(1), 25-32. doi:10.1089/acm.2006.6196.

Winkelman, M. (2003). Complementary therapy for addiction: "Drumming out drugs". *American Journal of Public Health, 93*(4), 647-651.

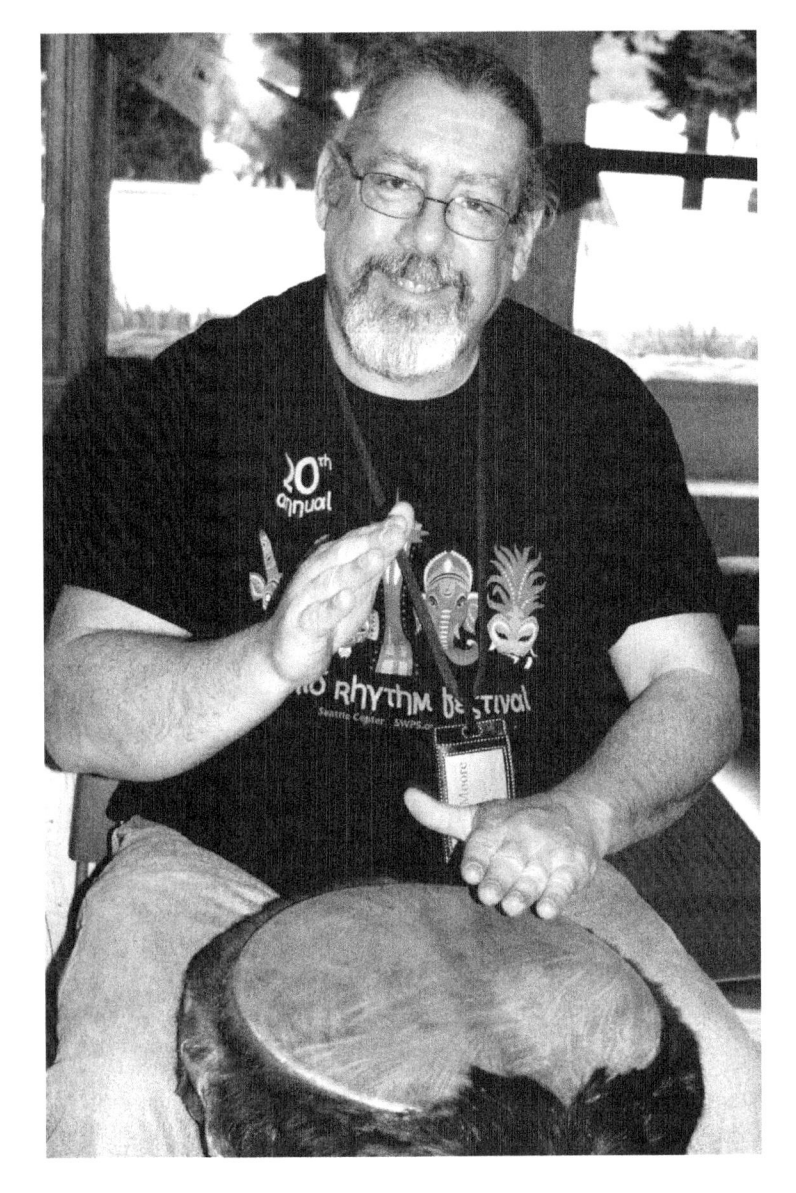

Contact Information

www.Outlawdrummers.com

Bill@outlawdrummers.com

Printed in Great Britain
by Amazon